FIT 4
The Master

Help To Overcome
Weight Loss Obstacles

SHELA A BROWN

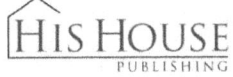
HIS HOUSE
PUBLISHING

Cover layout and design:
Tarsha L. Campbell
Dominionhouse Publishing & Design, LLC
www.mydominionhouse.com

DEDICATION

I would like to thank several people: I want to begin by thanking God whose mercy kept me until I decided to work with Him in this endeavor. I would like to thank my editors Karen & Judy for enduring my initial draft and working with me to get this message out. I would like to thank my sons, Lewis for being so gracious when the house became Oreo-free and Charles for expressing his frustration when I ate all the rice cakes. I especially thank my husband – Chester. I didn't know what this journey was going to be like. I merely asked you not to say anything. I asked you not to say anything regarding the food I bought. I asked you not to say anything regarding what you saw me eat. I asked you not to ask any questions about meetings I attended or conversations I had with people on the phone. I asked you to say nothing because I didn't want to feel like I was being watched. My dear Chester, your SILENCE was the greatest support and the greatest gift you could've ever given me... and because of that, I dedicate this book to you.

CONTENTS

Dedication

SECTION 1

My Story

Adding To My Faith

INTRODUCTION

People Magazine – January 2008 Issue

I don't normally buy magazines, but for some reason when I saw this one in the store, I picked it up. It was the issue that focused on people who had lost a lot of weight along with their before/after pictures. I remember looking at the photos. Several of the "before" pictures looked like me, women wearing sizes 24, 26, 28. I believe at that time I couldn't buy clothes in Marshall's or Ross anymore – the largest size they carried was a 24, which couldn't fit me. I wasn't sure if I wore a 26, 28 or even a 30 because I stopped caring. I just put on something to cover my body.

As I was looking through the pictures, I noticed they showed what they used to eat for lunch and what they ate now. One person used to eat McDonald's Super-size meal, extra double-cheese burger, and cookies for lunch. The "after" meals were things like a large salad with grilled chicken. The snacks that were once sodas, candy bars, and ice cream, now were fruit, protein bars, or nuts. I went to another person to see what they ate and their meals were similar.

No matter whose story I read when I looked at both meals, the "before" meal looked very similar to many meals I was eating at the time, and the "after" meal seemed strange. I cried a cry of despair! The idea of eating fresh vegetables, meat, and fresh fruit for one meal, much less for many meals, seemed so out of reach for me. I felt like a prisoner trapped in this obese body. The agony was extremely intense because deep down I knew I wasn't supposed to be this size, yet I felt trapped!

I've read enough information, heard enough unsolicited advice, and now the pictures were crystal clear in front of me. To get rid of these extra 100+ pounds I was carrying, I had to eat differently. Despair hit again! God, there is no way I… Me… Shela could possibly eat like this!!! I'm doomed!!! I closed the magazine feeling HOPELESS!!!

In my hopeless state, "God heard my despairing cry."

My Story isn't about a diet; it isn't about vitamins, minerals, cholesterol, antioxidants or any of those things (I don't know much about that stuff anyway). It is about my spiritual journey through a weight loss jungle. During this journey, I had to deal with not only the body issues (food desires, food preferences, and eating habits, etc); but I also had to deal with soul issues (emotions that I wanted to sedate with food); and spirit issues (situations that caused me to reach for food instead of God). As I dealt with these issues, I came to know God better – a lot better!

You will not find a particular diet in this book; neither will you find health tips, as that is not part of my story. However, you will find my experience of what I went through physically, emotionally and spiritually during the process of releasing over 100 pounds because for me, all three areas needed healing.

The outline of my story is taken from a scripture in the Bible, 2 Peter 1:5-8 (KJV).

*"And besides this, giving all diligence, **add to your faith** virtue; and to virtue knowledge; and to knowledge temperance; and to temperance patience; and to patience godliness; and to godliness brotherly kindness; and to brotherly kindness charity. For if these things be in you, and abound, they make you that ye shall neither be barren nor unfruitful in the knowledge of our Lord Jesus Christ."*

As I mentioned before, I believed deep down I was not supposed to weigh over 300 pounds; I was not supposed to wear sizes 26, 28 or 30. I was not supposed to breathe so heavy that when I spoke people were more concerned about my breathing than what I was saying. I believed I was supposed to be in a size 10/12 body. I believed I had a voice that influenced and encouraged, which could be heard better, with no breathing distractions. But there was something I had to add to what I believed, I had to…

ADD TO MY FAITH

ADD TO YOUR FAITH…
VIRTUE

Virtue! When I think of the word "virtue," the word "PURE" comes to my mind. Clean, Clear, and Untarnished. The TRUTH about where I am. No excuses, no cover ups, no explanations – the Truth… the PURE TRUTH about how I got to 300+ pounds. How I got myself to this point. What decisions did I make, what beliefs did I fall for, what instructions did I ignore that got me here?

Thanks to Facebook, people from my grammar school posted class pictures. I look at that little girl, and there is one thing I remember about her that was a common desire, wanting junk food and wanting "more" food. I wanted money so I could buy junk food or fast food. Having money to buy dolls or toys was not necessary. I just wanted money so I could buy penny candy, chips, candy bars, popsicles, ice cream cones, burgers, fries, and shakes. Occasionally I did want to buy a book. As the years went by the desires didn't change. I continued to primarily want money to buy junk food, fast food, and an occasional book.

Food held an unusual role in my life. My brother used to make jokes and say "Shela doesn't eat to live, she lives to eat." As people laughed, I remember thinking how true it was. The purpose for food in my life was not to keep me alive. The very idea of eating to live actually perplexed me. I didn't feel like I needed food to live; I needed food to do life. Then, food was a friend to me: potato chips, tortilla chips, candy bars, popcorn, cookies, donuts, muffins, macaroni & cheese, potato salad, candied sweet potatoes, french fries, rolls, cakes, pies, cobblers, ice cream… these were my friends. If I was bored, "my friends" kept me company. While I was in my office, my friends hung out with me. If my feelings got hurt, my friends helped me feel better. If I was mad, my friends were there to help justify my anger. If I was sad, my friends were there to console me. If I was happy, I called my friends to celebrate with me. If I was tired, my friends kept me awake (why I didn't just go to sleep still baffles me). If I was in an uncomfortable situation, as long as I could spot my friends in the room I was OK. If I was lonely, I looked forward to the company of my buddies. Actually, I enjoyed them even more when I was by myself because at those times

I didn't have to contend with open looks or comments of disapproval. Just me and my friends… *Aaah* heaven. Or so I thought.

As I got older, my weight climbed. To my knowledge, I never had blood pressure or cholesterol problems. But when my weight passed the 270-pound point, my knees started hurting and I had to start walking with a cane. One day, my sister-in-law saw me with my cane and said, "Shela, I don't like seeing you with that cane." She never said the words, but at that moment, I realized I was the fat lady with the cane. I soon learned how to walk without it but my knees still hurt. They continued to hurt to the point that I had to put away my 3 inch classic pumps. That was a sad day for me.

270 pounds is OK???

Oddly enough at 270 pounds, I told myself I was OK as long as I don't go past 275. So every day I weighed myself to make sure I wasn't over 275 pounds. My family went through a period where we lost everything. Our businesses, our income, our homes, our cars, our belongings… and we went into what I call a period of exile. During that time, I didn't care what I weighed. My mind just went blank to that aspect of my existence. Although I ignored the scale, I didn't ignore my "friends." When money was short, sometimes food was not available – I hated those days. I really needed my "friends" – and although money was slim, it was like I was in grammar school…my thought was "if I could just get some money to buy some chips, cookies or ice cream I would be OK." My weight continued to climb to over 300 pounds. At this stage, it took me 10 minutes to recuperate after walking up one flight of stairs and I usually gasped for breath just from walking 25 yards. It was at this time that I prayed my saddest prayer… at night as I lay down with my chest tight – "Dear God: for the sake of my children, please let me wake up tomorrow."

My "friends" were turning on me. They had been turning on me for quite some time but I enjoyed their company so much I didn't care. But now I started to care. The only problem was it seemed like it was too late.

Here's how I relate it to what the Apostle Paul said in Romans 7…

… I am… a slave to food. I do not understand why I eat like this, I want to eat right, yet I do not eat right. I hate how I eat, yet this is how I eat. I have a desire to eat better and take better care of my body, but I cannot do it. How I eat is not the way that is good for me. Even though I know it isn't good for me, I continue to eat like this anyway. Oh, the wretched soul of mine! Who can rescue me from this pathway to death?

AND TO YOUR VIRTUE ADD
KNOWLEDGE

Now that I had an untarnished perception regarding my view of food, I was clear about the knowledge I needed. I didn't need to get knowledge about diets, health tips, pills, juices or a garment. I needed to learn how to give food a different role in my life. But was that possible... for me???

Not knowing if it was possible, I remembered a message my Pastor's wife preached entitled "The Law of Relationships." She kept mentioning a scripture that referred to "... a brother has been raised for our adversity." Meaning, for every adverse situation in our life, God has raised someone else to help us. My mind went back to the *People Magazine*. These were people who used to eat just like I eat. But now they don't. I need to find one of these kinds of people.

Immediately I asked God, "please show me, let me meet the person and give me the courage to approach the person that is raised to help me with all this weight I am carrying." Let's be clear, I wasn't looking for a personal trainer or a health expert. I needed to find someone who had the same type of warped thinking I had, yet managed to lose over 100 pounds and was willing to walk me through how he or she did it.

Looking For Someone To Help

I was looking for someone who was 100+ pounds overweight and understood what it was like to eat in a manner that would lead to that amount of weight gain, even though it made no logical sense to keep doing so. I was looking for someone who understood the torment felt in amusement parks and airplanes because you weren't sure if the straps were long enough to buckle you in. I was looking for someone who understood what it was like not to know the last time they had a meal, because of the constant snacking, picking and bingeing on junk food. I was looking for someone who understood what it was like to have bags of frozen vegetables in the freezer that were over two years old. I was looking for someone who understood what it was like to be in the fruit and vegetable section of a grocery store and not know how to buy or how much to buy. I was looking for someone who knew what it was like to make several trips to the break room at work when no one was there and get more cake hoping no one saw you; so they won't realize you were the one that ate most of it. I was looking for someone who knew what it was like to view one serving size of chips as nothing shy of the entire bag, or a slice of pie to be nothing less than at least one-fourth of the pie. I was looking for someone who knew and understood all of this (and more) and still managed to lose over 100 pounds.

God reminded me of a fellowship I became aware of almost 20 years ago. I looked it up and found a meeting in my area. In those meetings, I found several people raised for this adversity. I listened to them. I listened to what they said they did. I listened to their stories. I listened to their hope. Their stories, their walk, their experiences and their faith gave me hope. People who were just the way I was. They were previously overweight, miserable, and both emotionally and spiritually numb. These people were not only 30, 50, 75, 90, 110, 220, 280 pounds smaller; they also had a message of hope. I could hear a connection to an aspect of God that I didn't know.

I went to the meetings every week. Every time I went, I learned more about me, more about my relationship with food and more about God. For the first few months, I was still eating the same way; but I kept going to the meetings. I kept adding knowledge. As I got more knowledge, my hope was restored. As my confidence was restored, I was coming to know God as a Healer. Healing my sick thoughts and healing my sick heart...

After a while, I came to realize food could no longer be my friend, my comfort or my ever present help. Food could no longer be what I reached for when I was down. Food could no longer be my redeemer or my savior. I remember hearing God say to me, "Shela if you ask Me to be a friend, a comforter, a present help, a redeemer, a savior – instead of expecting the food to be – I will."

One of the main things I noticed when I started attending these meetings was this: I had known God before I walked through those doors. I had a relationship with God before I walked through those doors. However, walking through those doors increased my knowledge and understanding of God. As He used the people and the spiritual principles of the program to grab me from the grips of despair, I came to know God as an amazing Redeemer. And because of the roles I allowed food to have in my life, I came to understand idolatry and experienced the love behind God's jealousy when we substitute other things for Him.

AND TO KNOWLEDGE ADD
TEMPERANCE

Temperance is not a word that prompts dreams, ideas, wishes, and hopes. It is a word that inspires ACTION. It was time to look at what I was believing for and add ACTION to it.

In the meetings I attended it is said, "Find someone in the room who has what you want and ask them how they are achieving it." I saw someone who had what I wanted and I decided to ask her how she did it. I listened to what she said. She didn't give me a diet. She only asked me to call her every morning. Tell her about what was going on in my day, tell her what I was going to eat that day, and ask God to help me to only eat what I planned – no matter what.

As simple as those steps were, I didn't do it the first day. Honestly, it took me a while to do those four things. She saw how difficult these simple tasks were and suggested we meet face-to-face to talk. Our discussion included a question: Am I willing to do what it takes to experience the benefits of normal eating or do I just want to reap the benefits while eating the way I wish to eat? My honest answer… I wanted to reap the benefits without doing the work. I wanted to reap the benefits by listening and feeling good about the work others were doing. And I wanted to reap the benefits by merely talking about the work that needed to be done. She, of course, let me know, "Shela, it doesn't work like that. Call me when you are willing to do the work." I left knowing I had a decision to make.

There is a phrase, "If you want something different you have to do something different." I'm sure most of us have heard some version of this phrase at least once or twice. Well, at some point it became necessary to take the knowledge I was getting from listening to those who already had what I wanted and do some of it myself.

That Sunday, one of the elders at church was talking about making a decision. Part of the word "decide" is the suffix "cide" which means to kill. When we make a decision something has to die. I realized at that point all of my excuses, preconceived notions and fears such as:

I don't want to eat the same thing all the time

I don't like healthy food

I don't like to cook

I can't afford to buy a lot of fresh fruit and vegetables

I can't think of healthy things to eat

I can't possibly go to a holiday dinner and not have ---

My fears of doing life without my "friends" – all these excuses and more had to DIE, if I was going to make a DECISION.

That night I was reminded of a scripture in Philippians, "… we are workers together with God." It hit me… I had to WORK WITH GOD.   I didn't make another promise to myself, "From now on, I'm not going to …" I simply prayed, "God, can you please help me to be willing to do what it takes to work WITH you. "

Saying Good Bye To My Friends

The next day I went to my job at the American Red Cross. The Mid-Florida Region Chapter has a great group of volunteers. They are so sweet and thoughtful. A large number of them must have been in a mood to bake the night before because that morning they brought lots of homemade baked goods for the staff.   In addition to a few of my "friends" in the vending machines, the kitchen was also filled with all of my favorite "friends" and even some new friends that looked and smelled delightful. I looked at the counter and screamed a prayer inside, "God, I can't walk away from this by myself. Please help me stay out of this kitchen today." I turned around, went back to my desk and worked.

People were coming by with the things they picked up. I prayed, "God, please help me stay out of that kitchen today" and I stayed in my seat. When the thought came to go and just look at what was in the kitchen I prayed, "God, please help me stay out of that kitchen today" and I stayed in my seat. When I had to pass the kitchen to go to the bathroom, I prayed, "God, please help me stay out of that kitchen today." I went to the bathroom and scurried back to my seat. At the end of the day I sat in my car bawling. Yet with much awe – God helped me to stay out of that kitchen. I had never walked away from my "friends." I certainly never walked away from my "friends" when they were free. And I definitely never walked away when everyone else was having some. But, that day I asked God to help me, and He did.

Someone said I stopped eating sweets cold turkey. That is not how I define that day. That day was not the day I stopped eating sweets cold turkey. September 8, 2008 was the day I made a decision to turn my will and life to the care of God to be my Friend, my Help, my Redeemer and Savior instead of turning my will and life to the care of a lemon tart.

I called the lady from the meeting and told her, "I'm ready to do what it takes." I talked to her or emailed her every day. I told her what was going on for the day, what I planned to eat and asked God to help me to eat what I planned. Most days I had to ask Him several times a day, but every time I asked Him, He came through.

As I continued to attend the meetings and listen to what others were doing, there was a standard message of having a plan for your food before the day began. I decided to follow that pattern.

I was given writing assignments. These assignments helped me to discover that when I ate certain foods it was harder for me to stick to my food plan. This was a gauge for me to eliminate foods or ingredients from my meals so I could have a victorious day. These assignments also pointed out some aspects of my behavior which made it harder for me to stick to my food plan. For example, if I exercised temperance by putting my food on a plate instead of using my fingers to eat out of containers and bags, or eating straight from the pot or refrigerator – it was surprisingly much easier to stick to my food plan.

Years ago I used to hear people say, "If you want to lose weight you need to just put down the fork." The contrary was true for me; if anything, I needed to pick up a fork and put down the hand-to-mouth motion.

As I continued listening to the experiences of others and followed suggestions and instructions given to me, I was adding temperance to knowledge and was having more and more days of victorious eating.

I found each time I set my food affections on "things above," which for me was a food plan I received from above (instead of setting my affections on what I felt like, what I was in the mood for, what others were having, or even what day the calendar said) I had a victorious day.

By having a plan for eating ahead of time, I don't have to make choices when I'm in a tempting situation. My food plan is my way of escape. It is a combat for what I termed the spirit called "More." That's the spirit that says stuff like, "Oooh that was good, I want some more," "Okay this is my last one," "For real, this is it, no more."

My plan says 3-4 oz of protein as part of my lunch meal is sufficient fuel for my body to carry out God's will for the day. Anything more than that is me appealing to my flesh.

Others have shared that in their experience, the amount of protein, vegetables, fruit, grain and dairy needed to carry out God's will for the day, doesn't change because it's a holiday, wedding, family gathering, social gathering or office party. I adopted that principle and found it to be easier to stay on the food plan/temperance wagon than it is to get back on the wagon.

My food plan is what I believe to be a prescription from God as to what I need to eat for the day to sustain my body to have the strength for the day and to have/maintain the body size God wants for me. Following my food plan is how I add temperance to the knowledge I receive.

AND TO YOUR TEMPERANCE ADD
PATIENCE

Adding patience. I remember Election Night 2008. Not just because of the election itself, but it was a night I was ready to say "forget it." I was two months on the plan and since the first week I'd lost 12 pounds, losing 28 pounds in 2 months didn't seem like it was good enough. You see although my head knew it was mostly water weight, I was still the fat lady on the bus. People at work were complimenting a girl who had been exercising for three months on how good she looked and no one noticed me. No one made a comment to me about my weight loss. So at that time I thought, "Why bother, I will always be the fat lady." I remember journaling I was afraid that I would never lose 50 pounds, 75 pounds, much less more than 100 pounds.

Fortunately, I kept listening to other people who had done or were also doing what I was trying to do. I kept doing what I did the day before. I added patience and kept doing what I did the day before. Combining patience with my temperance (a food plan) was about continuing to do what I did the day before regardless of how I felt about the progress. When I look in retrospect, twenty-eight pounds in two months is a lot and has no basis to ignite a fear of not losing more. At that moment, the enemy of my faith wanted me to throw in the towel. Had it not been for the people God raised for this adversity, I probably would have. I thank God for using them. I just added patience.

Patience…
Even With The Number On The Scale

To my temperance, I also had to add PATIENCE to consistently follow my food plan when I saw realistic results. I had to add PATIENCE when the scale moved 4 pounds in a month and I heard people around me talk about a special diet where you lose 20 pounds in a month. I had to add PATIENCE when I went to the store and saw pills that could boost weight loss by 50% (small print filled with questionable side-effects). I had to add PATIENCE when the temptation to abandon what I know is right for me and instead try a "quick fix." Especially at those times – I had to add patience to the act of diligently following my plan. When my weight only dropped 2/10 of a pound in one month, I had to add patience. When my weight reached a plateau for eight months, I had to add patience.

As I added patience to my temperance, Jehovah Shalom became real to me. I came to know PEACE.

FIT 4 The Master

AND TO YOUR PATIENCE ADD
GODLINESS

For this one to make sense, you have to remember the roles "my friends" played. If I was lonely, angry, hurt, disappointed, tired, irritable, frustrated, overwhelmed, happy, excited – I reached for "my friends" to get me through the emotion. Actually, it was more to sedate the emotion. Well, now I wasn't reaching for ice cream, popcorn or second helpings of macaroni & cheese.

My food plan was my guide for eating. But my food plan didn't stop the emotions from coming. What was I to do when I was angry with my husband, disappointed by a "NO" when I was expecting a "YES," irritated by leaders at church, fed up with my boss, overwhelmed by responsibilities, depressed about not having enough money to feed my children, buy Christmas presents or even to buy tampons? I was told to pause and keep pausing until I saw GOD higher than these situations. Anything shy of that, many times had me standing in the refrigerator with the door open looking inside. Even if I didn't pull anything out – that was always a dangerous place for me.

My mentor from the meetings always asked me what was going on in my day. She and others knew it was the activities of my day that would cause me to pick up something that was not part of my plan. No matter what I told her, she always followed it with the question – Where is God in that?

Some days I struggled with that question until I heard my pastor reference that particular beatitude in a message – "Blessed are the pure in heart, for they shall see God." His paraphrase was -- "If I have a pure heart, I will see God."

News Flash – Salty Crunch Snacks Don't Calm Me Down

I remember a time when I wasn't having a great day. I was extremely agitated and frustrated about some of the things I had to deal with for the day. In my mind, if I could just snack on something salty and/or crunchy, I would calm down and be able to make some sense of things. A friend of mine from my meetings warned me, "Shela that's the worst thing you could do. Whatever your next planned meal is, eat that and pray." It was almost time for my next meal, so I did that. Might I add, it took everything in me to focus only on putting the things I had originally planned to eat on my plate, and nothing more. No nibbling, no extra – just what I planned and the amount I planned. Once I finally had that plate prepared, I ate lunch and my prayer was simply – "God, please help me with today." After my meal and prayer, the anxiousness and agitation subsided and I was able to deal with the matters of the day with a clear and sound mind.

Adding godliness says when I am hurt, angry, overwhelmed, anxious, agitated, or irritated, I don't add fat-free pretzels, low-fat popcorn, baked chips or sugar-free popsicles - I add God! When my heart was pure of excess food, I could see God. And I found that if I seek Him, instead of something creamy, salty or crunchy I will find Him… especially if I seek HIM with all of my heart.

When I started to add godliness to patience, I came to know the God who is always there.

FIT 4 The Master

AND TO GODLINESS ADD
BROTHERLY KINDNESS

Sometimes people, institutions, policies or organizations got on my last nerve. They still do. Especially when it seems like my money, relationships, security or self-esteem is threatened.

Jesus said, if we confess OUR part, He is faithful to forgive and cleanse us from unrighteousness. When I am irritated with someone, I am usually rehearsing what they did wrong. If they did something, it takes me a while to get to the point of owning my part.

It was suggested to me that I revisit things in my past. Revisit them by looking briefly at what other people did, but concentrating more on my part. What was my part in the situations that had me irritated/angry/resentful/offended with my husband, my children, my parents, my siblings, my friends, my boss, my church leaders, school systems, protocols, banking systems, etc?

As I continued to practice focusing on my part and confessing my part, my heart was pure and I saw God much clearer in these situations. When I saw God, I also saw some act of kindness to add. I started with the act to pray for them. Praying that the good plans God has for their lives would happen for them was a must. Another act of kindness to add was forgiveness. Truth be told, a lot of times there was something about them that was also in me. So as I forgave them, I too, had an opportunity to acknowledge things about myself and ask for forgiveness. There were times when I had to do more than pray and forgive but I also had to do some other type of action that would bring about reconciliation. I'm still working on these, but I always ask God to help me to be willing to reconcile where I have hurt others.

Work Towards Living At Peace With All Men

God desires that we live at peace with all men. I understand that desire. When there is resentment, jealousy or fear, I am not at peace. When I'm not at peace, I want to reach for food to sedate my emotions. But when there is nothing in the air between another person and me, there is no need to sedate and I am able to be genuinely kind to God's people. When I encounter people that aren't acting perfectly, I remind myself of my imperfections and add brotherly kindness.

For real, for real – I work on this every day! I don't have it mastered, but it's getting better. As I listen to others and I self-reflect, I will continue to work on brotherly kindness and all of the other areas, every single day… one day at a time.

FIT 4 The Master

AND TO BROTHERLY KINDNESS ADD
LOVE

And now I add love and compassion for people. I love and care enough to share my experience with someone else who might be in despair. I love and care enough to walk someone through their journey, like someone did with me. I love and care enough to package what I have learned and give it to someone else. I love and care enough to stick to my food plan so someone else can see that they can too.

I was scared to share my story, much less to put it in print. I was afraid because I didn't think you wanted to hear what I had to say, or what if I gain weight or what if you criticized my story? Well, I finally asked God to remove any fears I had and help me to be who and what He wants me to be. Help me to be the person who loves enough to share a message of hope for those people who said the words, "Shela, how did you do it?" But the sound of the question reflected the pain of someone in prison.

I share my story as an act of love to that student, mother, professional, pastor's wife, evangelist, believer, that person who is suffering because they are locked up in a body (or a situation) they don't know how to get out of.

SECTION 1 CONCLUSION

IF THESE THINGS BE IN YOU AND ABOUND... you shall no longer be barren or unfruitful...

I have these before/after pictures here to show what God can do with a surrendered heart that is willing to work with Him. What you see below is the Lord's doing and it is marvelous in my eyes every time I look in the mirror. As God is helping me to add virtue, knowledge, temperance, patience, godliness, kindness and love – the more I abound in these, what I believed for (regular size body, a voice that isn't distracted by gasps) is not barren or unfruitful and my knowledge of Him is also not barren or unfruitful.

If reading this book reproduces a fruitful miracle in your life, then I am extremely grateful to God. Thank you for taking the time to read my story. I pray it is a source of encouragement for you and I pray it causes you to want to know God better.

God Bless You.

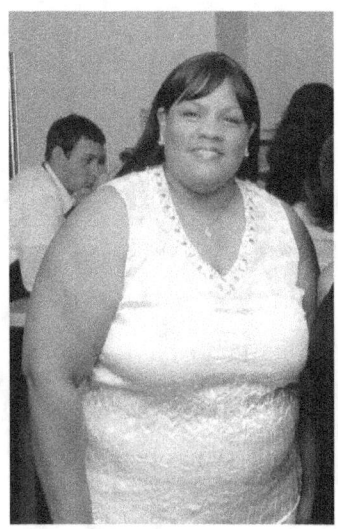
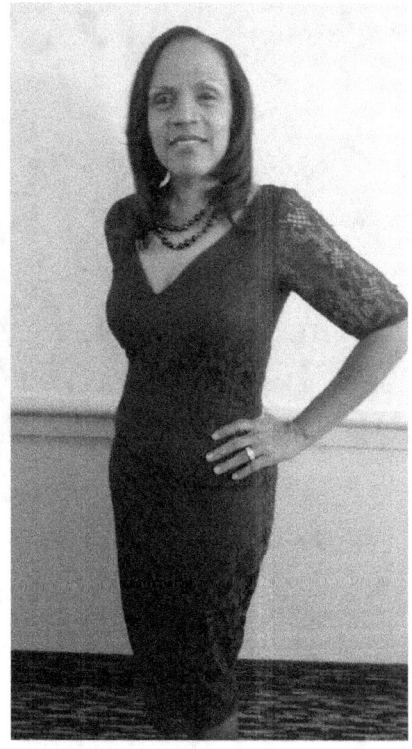

SECTION 2

His Strategy

OVERCOMING THE WEIGHT LOSS STRUGGLES

INTRODUCTION

Here I was. Two years after I released the first edition under the title "Add To Your Faith". Still maintaining the weight I loss +/- 10 pounds.

Then changes started happening. Routines began to change. Times of the meetings were no longer convenient, and some of the locations changed. But I was OK. I can handle this. I'll be fine. I know what to eat and what not eat. I'll be just fine.

So I started walking this journey alone. Life events occurred. Events causing a lot of personal anger, resentment and frustration. Job failures, business failures, financial crisis, deaths and much more happened. It was a season that brought me to my knees and on my face before God. In this season, I needed help not just with food but with life.

Even though my prayer time increased, I had no accountability for how I was eating, my portions increased, and my meals started to change. What started off as an extra piece of fruit because I had a "taste for something", turned into the entire cluster of grapes, or 2-3 extra apples. I told myself "it's fruit so it's OK." What started off as 1 bag of peanuts from the vending machine, turned into 2-3 bags of peanuts every day along with an occasional pack of peanut butter crackers and then several bags of baked potato chips. I told myself "it's not cookies so it's not that bad." Eventually french fries (aka potatoes fried style) and fried chicken (without the skin to keep it healthy) and wheat or multi-grain bread became regular items in my meals and they started to show up in between my meals. Slowly but surely when I wanted to relax, when I was bored, when I was nervous or afraid, I was mindlessly and impulsively eating. I was eating whatever I was in the mood for, with no plan. And although I was not eating sweets, I still gained 30 pounds of the 125 that I previously lost. My size 14 clothes couldn't fit. Since there was so much shame, there were no current profile pictures or selfies on Facebook (I kept reposting pictures from the previous year). I was gaining weight, fitting in size 16 and XL, hiding in shame, filled with remorse and eating an excess of "healthy food" to numb the pain.

But I believe God honored my time in prayer. By seeking Him, spending time with my Father – He protected me. I never did start eating sweets again – I believe a spirit of defeat would've come over me so intense, that I would not have recovered.

"In those days when you pray, I will listen. If you look for me wholeheartedly, you will find me. [14] I will be found by you," says the Lord. "I will end your captivity…" Jer 29:12 -14a NLT

I believe because of the prayers, He brought me to the cookie aisle in the grocery store. On this day, the cookies were talking to me. I looked at them - Chips Ahoy specifically. Then I went to the bakery department and gazed at the different cakes and pastries. Then I went back to the cookies aisle. I went back and forth about 2-3 times. Finally, as I was staring at the cookies, thinking I would just put them in my basket. All of a sudden I heard my Father /God say, "Shela don't let the devil punk you out like this. He wants to take you out – and this is how he wants to do it. Don't be fooled."

I tell people all the time, my weight loss is by the help of God. I think they believe I am just spiritualizing it. But I assure you, if it were up to me – on that day, those cookies would've been in my basket, in my car and half the pack would have been gone by the time I got home. And all night I would have been wrestling with the guilt of eating the cookies and strategizing on how to get to the car to eat the rest, all at the same time. BUT GOD STEPPED IN. This is how God helps me. He helps me to SEE and recognize the works of Satan. With those words I left the aisle, paid for my groceries and went to my car.

When I got in my car, I thought about those words. "Shela, don't let the Devil punk you out like this..." It dawned on me, the devil actually has an intentional agenda to punk me out. I heard the words again, "Don't let the Devil punk you out."

There is a devil, trying to punk us out, and it has a name. Its name is GLUTTONY, and it is a spirit that has resided in me for so long that I would not have recognized it, had God not revealed it to me as clearly as He did. Its agenda is to sabotage the God ordained projects, purposes, and assignments in me.

Gluttony, as it relates to food, is not just overeating, eating unhealthily and eating when you are not hungry but it is a demonic spirit with odd eating habits, compulsions, and cravings. When it is denied food or being denied certain types or amounts of food that it is craving – it will cause its victims severe emotional, mental or even physical distress.

This spirit fantasizes about food all the time. It uses food as a motivation and reward. It uses food to mask problems and as an escape. It uses food as a refuge for being sad, lonely, nervous, fearful or stressed out about financial, health, and relationship problems.

Gluttony traps its victim into thinking eating is helping them to be happy. It produces happiness at first and then FORCES the victim to continue going to food for happiness. But what the victim fails to realize is that the happiness they found the first few times is no longer available. Yet the victim is forced to continue going to food for happiness that is never found.

Sadly, gluttony is one of the most ignored demonic spirits in the church today. It has been ignored for so long that it has taken a position of tenure as if it legally belongs there.

While being ignored, it is adding fuel to the oppression and pain in the pews, among worship teams, admin staff, ministry leaders, pastors, first ladies, bishops and yes even five-fold presbytery.

While being ignored, it is given the freedom to forge ahead with its primary agenda of sabotaging God ordained purposes, assignments, relationships, organizations, and destinies. Thus causing its characteristics to almost seem normal. Characteristics like:

- Eating when we're not hungry
- Eating binges for no reason
- Thinking/strategizing about ways to get food in general or a particular food

- Planning ways to binge without anyone knowing
- Unable to stick to a diet
- Hidden anger when people talk to you about having willpower
- Can't stop eating certain types of foods even though our health is deteriorating
- Can't stop eating even though we want to

It will even cause its victim to get upset when reading this book because it knows it has been found out. (If that's you I urge you to keep reading... Trust the God you know and love and keep reading... Trust the God who knows and loves you and keep reading.)

The other unfortunate thing about its lengthy tenure is, we think it is part of who we are. We believe that this is the way it has to be. BUT I believe like myself, there are some who see themselves constantly eating when they didn't want to. Then there are some who are thinking about how they can get more food without people noticing, and then others who feel enslaved to food – yet through the promptings of the Holy Spirit, there is a still small voice that tells them, "This is not normal, life does not have to be like this, I can be free. I don't know how, but I know I can be free."

For those who sense and believe that, I am here to declare,

"we can be free!" This is not of God! God does not want us to be enslaved to this. The schemes and strategies to plan a food binge do not reflect a mind that is in Christ Jesus. We can be free from this and God desires to set us free. It is possible for food just to be food. It is possible for food to just sustain us - period. It is possible to eat a meal and continue being about the Father's business. It is possible and the Good News is God wants that for us.

We start the process of becoming free by recognizing its existence. Understanding the effect it has in our lives and recognizing its tactics.

The language in the meetings I told you I attended, would call temptations and irrational suggestions to eat, "a disease." They would say, "It was our disease talking." I never could embrace that because when I think of a disease, I think of sicknesses, ailments, infections and viruses. This was not a disease. What was happening inside of me was more than that. This was something that had an agenda. It had a structured plan. Although it appeared as though I was eating whatever I was in the mood for with no rhyme or reasoning, this was its precise methodology. It had a goal to steal, kill and destroy my dreams, my purpose, my esteem, my assignment. And that is not the characteristic of a disease, that is how my Bible defines SATAN – the DEVIL. And if we resist the Devil, he will flee. Continuing to ignore this devil will not make him flee. Continuing to ignore this devil will allow it to fulfill its primary agenda, and that is to steal, kill and destroy the purpose God has trusted you with. I urge you, don't let God down – not over a piece of cake, loaded burrito or chili cheese fries.

It is time to lay aside the weight and lay aside the sin of gluttony that so easily trips us up.

In light of the price Jesus paid for us, it is time to present our bodies as a living sacrifice, holy and acceptable to Him. This is the least we can do.

2 Tim 2:21 NLT says, "One who cleanses himself from these things will be a vessel for honor, sanctified, fit for the Master's use, and prepared for every good work."

It is time to prepare our vessels to be FIT 4 The Master's use, prepared for every good work. It is time to use a strategy to daily kick the Spirit of gluttony out of my life. Despite its tenure, it has no legal right to reside in me, influencing my decisions on how to eat. But because most trespassers don't leave until the owners exercise their legal authority – this spirit of gluttony is not going anywhere until we kick it out!

The Bible tells us, if "we resist the devil he will flee from us." This is a strategy that will build our resistance on a daily basis so this devil will flee and will finally be evicted from the areas it is trespassing in; areas both known and unknown to us.

Let's be clear. We are not talking about a diet! There is more at stake here. This is more than the number on a scale and more than the size of clothing. We are talking about the purpose and assignment God has entrusted us with. This is spiritual warfare! The weapons of our warfare are not carnal, but they are mighty through God in pulling down STRONGHOLDS. The weapons of our warfare are mighty enough to pull down every STRONGHOLD that told us to accept as unchangeable, situations like our body size and health conditions that we know are contrary to the will of God.

With that, I'd like to introduce you to...

The FIT 4 The Master Strategy

FIT 4

THE MASTER STRATEGY
FOLLOW A FOOD PLAN

"Commit everything you do to the Lord.
Trust him, and He will help you"   Psalm 37:5 NLT

Food plans provide specific boundaries. I find it to be a lifestyle of fasting, which is necessary to break the physical, psychological and emotional addiction or attraction to excess food. It is arduous and as we remain committed over an extended period of time, it is common to experience some slips and disappointments along the way. This is why we do not do it alone and it is also why after we have recovered; additional strength comes by restoring a brother.

I am not an advocate of a specific plan. I believe as Christians, we are to be led by the Spirit. God our creator knows how we are to eat to accomplish what He created us to do. If we allow Him, He will lead us to a plan for eating.

Over the years, my food plan has changed, primarily because I was being led by the Spirit. There were a few occasions when it changed because I was led by my flesh. Those did not bring favorable results. My flesh kept asking for more and there was an inner restlessness. Even when changes to my plan were to satisfy my flesh, because of my commitment to follow the plan, God remained faithful in leading me. He led me to several mentors that required me to follow their plans. He led me through information from nutritionists. He led me many times by conviction. The Holy Spirit will guide you to what is needed for you to be able to work together with God.

Once the Holy Spirit leads you to a food plan, unless there is a medical reason to change it, stick with it for a period of time. Do not change it to the latest thing that promises to help you lose weight faster. Trust the plan God guides you to. This is not about the latest diet. This is about becoming FIT 4 The Master's purpose and assignment for your life.

If you want to change the plan, remember there really is a lot of safety and protection from gluttony with counsel. The times I made changes without counsel, I found myself making more and more changes that "made sense to me." And because a fool is wise in his own eyes, before I knew it, the number on the scale went up and my clothes became very tight. To put it bluntly, the last time I made a series of changes to my food plan, I eventually gained 30 pounds. Again, there is much safety from the spirit of gluttony with counsel.

How to find a Food Plan?

As I looked for a food plan to follow on a regular basis, I looked for someone else who previously struggled with similar symptoms and asked them what they did and what they ate. More often than not, I found a person who needs to lose 10 or 20 pounds can approach food differently than a person that is 75, 100, 150+ pounds overweight.

So get assistance from someone else that has been on this journey longer then you. Fast, pray and ask God to direct you to a plan that will help you to be FIT 4 His use. Do not delay. PRAY. Make a decision TODAY to start on a plan and believe the Holy Spirit will guide you. Go ahead and make your grocery list – according to a specific food plan and make a decision to FOLLOW the Plan.

Examples of plans I've been on are in the back of the book.

I also recommend starting off with a Plan that could also be a Fast. An example would be 30 days on…

The Fit 4 The Master Break Through Food Plan

Breakfast:
3-4 oz protein, 4-6 oz fruit

Lunch:
3-4 oz protein, 6-8 oz raw vegetables, 6-8oz cooked vegetables, 4-6 oz fruit, 1 T fat

Dinner:
3-4 oz protein, 6-8 oz raw vegetables, 6-8oz cooked vegetables, 4 oz starch or grain, 1 T fat

No Sugar, No Flour, No Artificial Sweetener, No Caffeine

This Plan declares we are <u>Breaking Through</u> into a New Way of Eating. It is designed to starve things our flesh desires so we can be sensitive to how the Spirit wants to lead us in our eating. During the 30 days, we ask God for wisdom on how to recognize the plan He wants for us and we ask Him to give us the grace to receive the instruction He provides. During these 30 days we surrender our eating habits, beliefs and desires to our loving Father.

The plan I am on today is not the plan I was on when I started. The Holy Spirit guided me through several plans, because He knew I couldn't handle the plan I'm on today, when I first started. So trust the process the Holy Spirit leads you through.

F**I**T 4

THE MASTER STRATEGY
INTERACT WITH THE WORD

"In those days when you pray, I will listen If you look for me
wholeheartedly, you will find me. I will be found by you," says the Lord.
"I will end your captivity…"   Jer 29:12-14 NLT

GLUTTONY is a sin of the flesh, and the flesh opposes the Spirit. Not only does gluttony manifest in weight gain, illnesses and slowly wearing down our bodies, it also slowly eats away at our hunger for God. Our daily time in the presence of God slowly dwindles to days and even weeks or dare I say months of no quality time with the Father. No quality time with God drains us and keeps us foggy in the head. The reconciliation to God that Jesus died for becomes so elusive that there is now something blocking us from the Father.

This interaction is not the time we spend to prepare for the next message, Bible Study, or Sunday School lesson. It is also not the time we spend just to say we read the Bible today. It is more than that.

We are spending time interacting with the Word. The word "act" is the process of doing. So when we INTERACT with the Word, we go through the process of doing something with the Word, AND we allow the Word to go through the process of doing something with us. Interacting with the Word is having a heart connection with the Word.

A mentor of mine uses a phrase "BIBLE IMMERSION." We IMMERSE ourselves in the Word by reading, underlining passages and phrases that stand out. This is going through the process of doing something with the Word. But we don't stop there, we then let the Word go through the process of doing something inside us, we pause long enough so the Word can reach our heart. This is done by meditating on the passages, writing on those passages and praying what God reveals to you through the passage. With this, we are allowing God to reveal His thoughts toward us through His Word.

When we interact with the Word on a daily basis we will

see that the Word really is powerful enough to heal our souls, our emotions, thoughts, desires (yes even our food desires), imaginations and intellect in the areas that the spirit of gluttony ransacked.

As I interacted with the Word, there were many times I read a chapter or two and received nothing. But as I prayed for something in what I read to penetrate my heart, and then paused, every single time the Holy Spirit lit my heart and revealed something in the passage that interacted with something in my heart.

Let's be clear about something, the enemy wants us to think that interacting with the Word of God, has nothing to do with how we eat. And to the intellectual mind; it seems like it doesn't. Except, we're actually not dealing with food. This is bigger than eating right. How we eat is simply a symptom of other things going on in our lives. Interacting with the Word will bring the light of God, the healing power of God and the love of God to those things. Our health, eating habits and body size are also symptoms of a stronghold which can be broken as we hear and hear and hear the Word.

So we have to believe that the Word we are reading will work. For a period of time, I had to consciously remind myself and DECLARE that the Word I was reading today, really was alive and powerful. The Word I was reading today was cutting between spirit and soul. The word I was reading at that very moment - regardless of the text - was exposing innermost thoughts and desires. I had to believe the Word I was reading was delivering me from the ways the enemy wanted to destroy my life. I had to believe the Word that reached my heart really did have enough power to save my soul. The Word that entered my heart was POWERFUL enough to save/rescue my thoughts, emotions, desires, intellect, and imagination. I had to believe and declare that the Word I was reading TODAY was working in my life – specifically in my eating habits.

FI **T** 4

THE MASTER STRATEGY
Touch Others In Agreement

"I also tell you this: If two of you agree here on earth concerning anything you ask, my Father in heaven will do it for you. For where two or three gathers together as my followers, I am there among them." Matt 18:19-20 NLT

You have heard me say many times; I have not been able to walk this journey successfully alone. So when I read this text, my spirit jumps and gets excited because I lived and experienced the truth in this. When I am in agreement with someone else concerning being free from the ways food and gluttony entraps me, my Father is in the midst of it. When I gather with a few more people that are trying to follow Jesus in this area of their life; GOD IS IN THE MIDST. And when God is in the midst, on my worst day the devil can only go so far.

So we must make a conscious effort to bring God in the midst. On our own and by ourselves we are at high risk of being defeated. When I retreat or isolate, when I decide I don't feel like talking to anybody, when I feel like I don't need to connect with anyone, when I decide I know what to do so "I got this," when I tell myself I don't want to bother anyone ... I put myself in jeopardy of being blindsided by hits because the enemy has me alone. Touching, connecting/talking with others that agree with being committed to living a life of victory in this area, brings God into the midst and when He is in the midst -- the devil ain't got a chance!

This is a spiritual battle. It is not about a diet. We need GOD! We need GOD's help. We NEED GOD to be IN THIS WITH US! I said it before and I'll say it again when I say "God helped me" that is not a cliché. So many times, when the temptation and the urges were so intense... God helped me through the testimony, witness, knowledge, encouragement and sharing of others who are also warring with this spirit.

Touching by way of talking or connecting with someone

else or by way of attending a group meeting with others in agreement also brings reinforcement. Deut 32:30 says "how could one person chase a thousand of them, and two people put ten thousand to flight… unless the Lord had given them up?"

The Spirit of Gluttony has been whispering, suggesting, giving advice for so long – we sometimes are not able to recognize its tactics on our own. Even though we have the authority to command it to leave, we may not be aware of its hiding places or invitations. Consequently, we've extended opportunities for it to return. So the reinforcement of the 2nd person can help us recognize its presence and can help us detect its suggestions and influences.

This support helps us understand the tactics of the spirit of gluttony. In the past, it has EASILY BESET US… We need support so that it is not so EASY to get us.

To some, the spirit of gluttony has been trespassing so long, we have embraced it as part of the family, and have gotten comfortable with the weight. We've decided this is the way it is. High blood pressure and diabetes run in the family so we've learned how to do life with it. The reinforcement helps to remind you that God wants something better for your life than frustration over tight fitted clothes, shame over the weight gain and sadness over ill health. The reinforcement reminds you that its tenure means nothing.

The reinforcement helps you to recognize the damage it is doing. The reinforcement is to help you see that you have a legal right to get rid of it. The reinforcement reiterates the GOOD that God has for you.

The reinforcement is also a resource of knowledge of living life free from gluttony. What do I do when I'm at an event where I would usually over indulge? I don't want to graze at the buffet table or dessert table all night, that isn't my desire – but I'm so use to doing that, what should I do now? The connection with others will give us wisdom on how to handle events. What do I do when life hits me with curve balls? The connection with others will allow us to hear testimonies that will build our faith.

Personally, I touch and connect with an accountability partner/mentor/sponsor and a community of believers.

My accountability partner/mentor/sponsor normally guides me in selecting a food plan and changing a food plan. Because I know this is an area that the devil wants to use to destroy my life, I keep what I do with food out in the open. I let that person know what I am going to eat or what I ate. No matter what it was. When I sneak what I'm eating, I open up the door for gluttony to trespass again. With that being said, I touch base with someone EVERY DAY via a telephone call, a text or an email about what I ate and what I'm going to eat. This works for me.

I also connect with a community of believers by way of participating in live meetings, telephone meetings or online groups. These groups are separate from my attendance and involvement in regular church meetings. These groups deal specifically with walking in victory in the areas of compulsive overeating and food addiction which are both manifestations of gluttony. There are companies of believers around the world, who press toward living in freedom every day. So yes, I deliberately touch and agree with those people, because this is a sin that can EASILY BESET ME.

By participating in these groups, I have also been able to find mentors for accountability and guidance with food plans. By taking part in the groups, I found a mentor to guide me with food plans. I develop relationships with people that I can call when I need suggestions, wisdom or words of encouragement.

The following websites have information about Christian recovery groups and telephone meetings. I am sure this is not an exhaustive list but these groups have been helpful to me.

christianfoodaddicts.weebly.com

bibleforfood.org

bible4recovery.com

fulloffaith.com

In addition to these, there is a FIT 4 THE MASTER Weekly Prayer Call for those struggling with losing weight. There is a FIT 4 THE MASTER Community you can join to receive encouragement and provide assistance. Also, there is a FIT 4 THE MASTER Strategy Session to personalize the strategy for your lifestyle and a FIT 4 THE MASTER Coaching Program to help you get started and to assist you while on the journey of losing weight. To sign up and/or get additional information on the ways FIT 4 THE MASTER can support you on this journey, visit our website – www.fit4themaster.com

As you participate in these groups, you will see there are programs within them to help address the issues that have given this spirit of gluttony access. Again, this is not about a diet – this is a spiritual issue, which needs a spiritual solution along with the food plan.

FIT 4

THE MASTER STRATEGY
4 GOOD THINGS

"This is the day that the Lord has made, I will rejoice and be glad in it." Psalm 118:24

If your flesh is responding in fear about what it has to give up and how it can't have certain foods anymore, let me assure you how normal that is. A very common tactic the enemy uses is to make you feel like you are going to be missing out on some excellent food or meal. He will have us believe giving up habits that are causing our health to deteriorate is the most dreadful thing we can do and the worst thing in the world. He will have us believe we aren't ready and can deal with this later. What he doesn't do is bring to our mind the many times we've cried out to God for help because we were distressed about test results or a doctor's prognosis or even the number on the scale that was gradually increasing. Nevertheless, in our pain- God heard our cry, and from His goodness, God responded to our cry.

Every day that the Lord has made, it is important to make a decision to rejoice and be glad in the things God is doing – specifically as it relates to His response to our cry for help. We have to acknowledge daily how good God is. As we put limits on foods and eliminate them, the enemy would love for us to feel like we are being deprived. When the truth is, these limits are giving us good things. They are giving us good health, good stamina, good clarity, good relationships, good days, good sleep and yes, right body/clothing size. And all these GOOD THINGS come from the Lord. These GOOD THINGS do NOT come from "poor me pity parties" that the Devil would like for us to waddle in, to drive us right back to the place of despair.

Grumbling and complaining about what we can or can't have, will have us as the children of Israel. Like them, we will be stuck in the wilderness wondering why we aren't getting better.

We have to take the time to think on at least **4** GOOD things that are happening as we are becoming and staying FIT

4 the Master. Honestly, I initially picked the number 4 because it flows with the title. But as I looked up the spiritual significance of the number 4, it is the number of God's creative work.

As we take steps into victory, God is creating so much good in our life. There are good works that God is creating as we follow the food plan He has given us through counsel. There are good works God is creating as we interact with His Word. There are good works God created as we touch and agree with others on this journey. As we acknowledge the good works He created, there will be a release of more good works that you will begin to see. So when the enemy causes you to think giving in to the influences of gluttony is GOOD, you will begin knowing without a shadow of a doubt, it is a LIE.

Every day that God makes, we have to combat the enemy by making a decision to rejoice and be glad in all the GOOD that God is giving us as we take victory steps.

2 Tim 2:20-21 NLT reads

In a wealthy home, some utensils are made of gold and silver, and some are made of wood and clay. The expensive utensils are used for special occasions, and the cheap ones are for everyday use. If you keep yourself pure, you will be a special utensil for honorable use. Your life will be clean, and you will be ready for the Master to use you for every good work.

I will remind you again, the agenda of the spirit of gluttony is to steal, kill and destroy the purpose that God has entrusted you with. I believe the enemy wants to reduce your purpose as something cheap for everyday use when God has special occasions in mind for you. I urge you, don't let God down. There are special occasions in your future for which the Master wants to use you.

Join me in getting FIT 4 The Master!

We're in this for the long haul because
The Master Has Need of Us

SECTION 2
CONCLUSION

I listened to the comments and reactions of those who read the first edition. I realized many recognized how food affected their physical health, emotional health, and spiritual health and they were asking for more.

So I have developed a community called The FIT 4 THE MASTER COMMUNITY. You can join the community by signing up on the Fit 4 The Master website or liking the Fit 4 The Master Facebook Page. (www.fit4themaster.com)

The Master has need of you. So join the Fit 4 The Master Community. This is a tough journey and you don't have to do it alone.

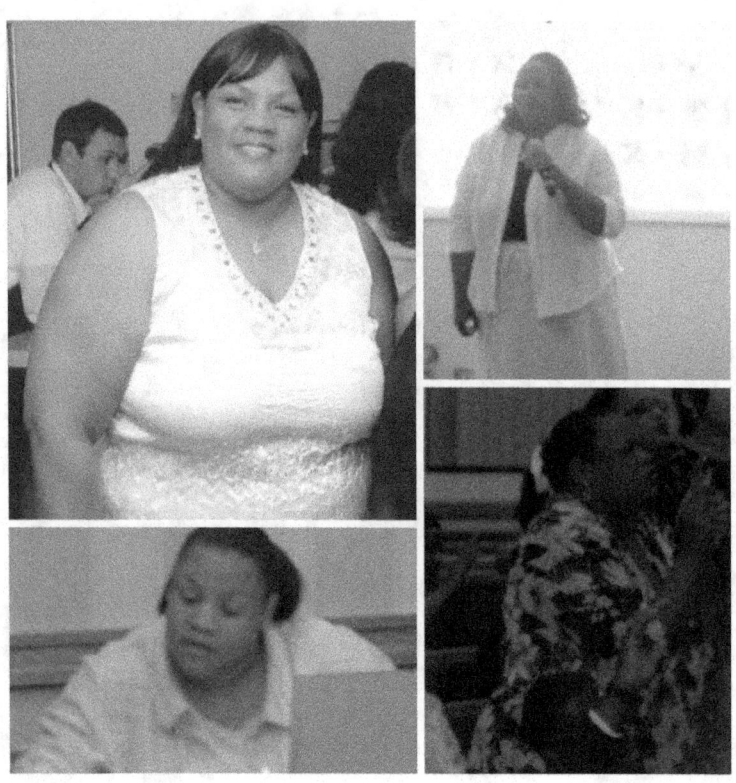

2005 – 2008

It was very hard to find "before" pictures of myself. I didn't like seeing myself in pictures so I avoided the camera. But these are a few of my most recent pictures before starting this journey

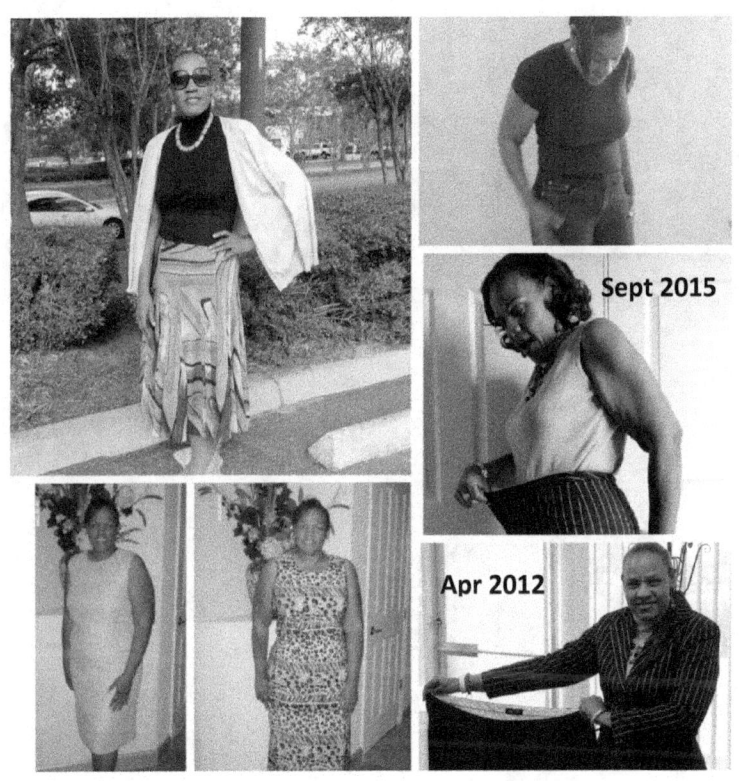

2009 - Present

Counter-clockwise, starting with bottom left
Progression for first 100 pounds (it took 14 ½ months).
A huge surprise came in Sept 2015, when my pants from Apr 2012
were now several sizes too big.
Top right is my first time wearing a size 10 jeans – my goal size

ABOUT THE AUTHOR

Overweight her entire life, Shela Brown began a journey to lose over 100 pounds at age 44. This was a scary endeavor for Shela because the last time she attempted to lose weight, she was in her twenty's. She lost 40 pounds but was only able to maintain it for two months. The next 18 years she was never able to stick to a diet long enough to lose weight and just continued to gain weight until she exceeded 300 pounds.

After decades of believing she could never be a smaller size, in Sept of 2008 Shela decided to try to lose weight one more time using an approach other than the latest fad diet or popular diet programs. This approach proved successful because on November 26, 2009 (Thanksgiving Day), Shela stepped on a scale and it was 100 pounds less than her highest weight.

Although her weight fluctuated for a few years, she still maintained the significant weight loss for several years. And when her weight loss plateaued in 2013, Shela had to make a few more adjustments to losing those last stubborn 30 pounds (pre-menopausal). Shela achieved her goal size 10 while writing the 2nd edition of her book (October 2015).

Now Shela is armed, dangerous and ready to release a sound and a message that will ignite hope, encouragement and victory to others still struggling with unwanted excess weight.

Shela Brown is married with two sons and currently resides in Central Florida. As an Author, Coach and Inspirational Speaker, Shela is available for book signings, speaking engagements and coaching and can be contacted by way of the following:

Contact Form on the website www.fit4themaster.com
Email at fit4themaster@outlook.com
Facebook at facebook.com/Fit4TheMastersUse.

JOIN THE
FIT 4 THE MASTER
COMMUNITY

- Like Our Facebook Page
  www.facebook.com/Fit4TheMastersUse

- Join Our Email List at
  www.fit4themaster.com

- Sign Up for a FIT 4 The Master Coaching
  Program
  Email Shela at fit4themaster@outlook.com

- Schedule a complimentary one on one FIT 4
  The Master Breakthrough Strategy Session
  Email Shela at fit4themaster@outlook.com

FIT 4 The Master

Examples of Food Plans I've Been On

Plan #1
Breakfast:

2 oz protein, 1 starch/grain serving, 1 fruit serving

1 cup milk or milk substitute

Lunch:

3 oz protein, 1 starch/grain serving, 1 fruit serving, 3 vegetable servings 2 fat servings

Dinner:

3 oz protein, 1 starch/grain serving, 1 fruit serving, 3 vegetable servings

2 fat servings

Bedtime:

1 starch/grain serving, 1 fruit serving, 1 cup milk/dairy or milk substitute

No Sugar (food where sugar is in the first 4 ingredients)

Plan #2
Three Meals a Day

Min 8 oz Veg for Lunch and Dinner

No in between snacks, bites, licks or tastes

No sugar or flour (food where sugar or flour is in the first 4 ingredients)

Plan #3
Breakfast:

4oz Protein, 1 fruit, 8oz dairy, 1 grain

Lunch:

4 oz protein, 8oz salad (raw veg) 8oz cooked veg, 1 fruit or 1/2cup starch, 1T fat or 2T salad dressing

Dinner

4 oz protein, 8oz salad (raw veg,) 8oz cooked veg, 1 fruit or 1/2cup starch, 1T fat or 2T salad dressing

Snack:

8oz dairy, 1 grain

No sugar or flour (food where sugar or flour is in the first 4 ingredients)

Plan #4
Breakfast:

4oz protein, 1 fruit, 4oz grain

Lunch:

4 oz protein, 8oz salad (raw veg,) 8oz cooked veg, 1 fruit, 1T Fat

Dinner:

4 oz protein, 8oz salad (raw veg,) 8oz cooked veg, 4-6oz raw veg, starch or grain 2T fat

No sugar or flour (food where sugar or flour is in the first 4 ingredients) No Artificial Sweeteners